ANXIETY NEUROSIS
Good Health with Yoga & Ayurveda

By Dr.Jacob.K.

©2019

Contents

DESCRIPTION 3

CHAPTER 1. WHAT ARE THE SYMPTOMS OF NEUROSIS? 1

CHAPTER 2. TYPES OF NEUROSIS 2

CHAPTER 3. AYURVEDIC MEDICINES WITH PROVEN EFFECTS 4

CHAPTER 4. SIDDHA MEDICINES USEFUL AND HELPFUL 5

CHAPTER 5. BEST 3 HOME REMEDIES FOR ANXIETY 6

CHAPTER 6. SINGLE HERBAL MEDICINAL PLANTS 7

CHAPTER 7. COMPOUND AND CLASSICAL AYURVEDIC FORMULATIONS 8

CHAPTER 8. YOGIC PRACTICES 10

CHAPTER 9. BENEFICIAL YOGA POSTURES 11

CHAPTER 10. IMPORTANT FOOD THAT CAN HELP REDUCE ANXIETY. 26

CONCLUSION 29

Description

Anxiety disorders or primarily known as Neurosis. Understanding neurosis is very essential. Its plural term is neuroses. People make a big mistake in these 2 terms of neurosis and neuroses. Neurosis is no longer used in medical practice. Neurosis is characterized by any emotional feelings of distress and moments of unhappiness depression or anxiety.

This may impair the persons functioning of his life, affairs, relationship. However not widely used neurosis diagnosis is essential to understand how some psychological disorders can be treated.

Neuroses is often misunderstood to neuroticism. Understanding the condition of the patient is very essential. Talking more about neuroticism it's never a short-term, neither it's a medical condition. It's a long-term tendency to be in a negative or an in an emotional anxious state.

Neuroticism affected people are very susceptible to environmental stress. They tend to suffer from guilt feeling, hatred, anger, anxiety, envy, as compared to other people. These people they tend to find everyday normal situations as major and they get worried and anxious about that. Some may even experience frustrations that can become a problem for them and which gradually leads to disparity. These people can be very shy and self-conscious, which results them into various types of phobias. Some of the phobias that an individual encounter are being negative, having an aggressive behaviour, panicking all the time, always in a depressive mood, tend to be anxious always.

People with anxiety disorders very often fall into addictions like drugs and other stimulants. If unchecked it can lead to partial paralysis, none functioning or abnormal functioning of the organs. May also result in sexual dysfunction.

Chapter 1. What are the symptoms of neurosis?

Individual suffering from neurosis often have bouts of envy anger guilt,
Feel very restlessness all the time , complains of mild to severe headache , feel nauseated, experience palpitations, nervousness, excessive sweating , feeling breathlessness , bad digestive system ,
Dysentery, increased heart rate. Disturbed sleep, lack of concentration, can't focus on things.
Anxiety disorders occur when a person regularly feels disproportionate levels of distress, worry, or fear over an emotional trigger. Identifying the reason behind a presentation of anxiety can be the key to successful treatment.
To assist diagnosis, the conditions under the umbrella of anxiety disorders have certain characteristics that set them apart from normal feelings of anxiety. A wide variety of factors can contribute to anxiety disorders.

Chapter 2. Types of Neurosis

There are different type of neurosis.
Anxiety neurosis- this neurosis is characterised by unwanted worry, extreme anxiousness, which can lead to the person ending up having panic attacks, excessive sweating and shivering.

Obsessive compulsive neurosis- this form of neurosis involves repetitive intrusive behavioural patterns, mental acts and thoughts which can distress the person.

Post-traumatic neurosis- Some past deep and brutal traumatic events causes stress and inability to function in everyday chores.

Compensation neurosis- covers all phobias

Depressive neurosis- this is characterized by long lasting apathy and reluctance towards any activity.

Hysterical neurosis- in this the patient theatrically exposes their problems.

The technical word meaning of neurosis is nerve disorder. Often mental illness is described as anxiety neurosis.

Excessive worry and stress leads to anxiety neurosis. This can give rise to physical conditions like shivering, nausea, sweating, and chest pain. The patient often feels claustrophobic. He or she will find it difficult to make a decision, always finds themselves in a confused state. More to add on to the most prominent symptoms. They are bouts of Palpitations, the body especially the hands and the legs tend to tremble and shiver, the patient may feel dizzy and may be have vertigo. There may be tingling sensation in the hands and feet (Paraesthesia). This could be a quite common symptom. Excessive perspiration especially on the palms and the forehead. There may be shortness of breath associated with mild chest pain. The sleep can be disturbed; it can also upset the digestive system which can cause loss of weight in an individual. In women suffering from anxiety the menstruation can be disturbed and irregular with hot and sold sensation throughout the body. Body feel lethargic with cold feet whilst your body could be sweating. In the episode of an attack the bottom lip can flicker continuously.

Chapter 3. Ayurvedic medicines with proven effects

Sharibadhi kwatham - 30ml thrice daily before food
Brihath Vathachinthamani Ras - 120mg twice daily with honey followed by the decoction of jatamansi
Aswagandhadhi Choornam - 3-6 gm twice daily with milk
Aswagandharishtam - 15-30 ml twice daily after food
Brahmi Gritham - 10gm at night with milk

Chapter 4. Siddha medicines useful and helpful

Vallarai Nei   -1-2 teaspoon thrice daily
Bhrami Nei   -8-15 ml once daily
Peranda Parpam   -100-300 mg with goats milk, ginger juice and crystal sugar.

Whilst taking the above medicines, try and avoid too much of spices, chilly and sour food.

Chapter 5. Best 3 Home remedies for anxiety

1. Grated fresh coconut 10gms, peeled and soaked almonds three in number, fennel seeds powdered 5 gms, black pepper powdered 2 gms, crystal sugar 20gms
Mix the above with milk which is formerly soaked in with 6 threads of saffron for 6 hours and drink it daily.
This home based remedy has helped to calm the nervous system.

2. Licorice root powdered 1 teaspoon with water to drink in the morning in empty stomach for 21 days.
This drink is a called as Medhya Rasayana in Ayurveda and it is considered to rejuvenate the mental health.

3. Fresh rose petals in a cup of boiling water. Let it get lukewarm, after it's lukewarm add half a teaspoon of crystal sugar to it and have it twice a day.
This is a very good drink to energise the body and cool the internal system.

Chapter 6. Single Herbal Medicinal Plants

Ashwagandha Powder (Withania somnifera) 3-5 gm along with sugar or clarified butter for 15 days. Twice a day before food.

Jatamansi Powder (Nardostachys jatamansi) 500 mg - 1 gm with milk twice daily after food for 15 days

Brahmi Powder (Bacopa monnieri Linn.) 2gms with water twice daily before food for 15 days.

Mandookaparni Powder (Centella asiatica Linn.) 2gms with water twice daily before food for 15 days

Chapter 7. Compound and Classical Ayurvedic Formulations

Kalyanaka ghritha — 1 teaspoon with warm milk twice daily before food for 15 days.

Brahmi vati — 500 mg with water twice daily before food for 15 days.

Sarpagandhadi vati — 125 mg with milk twice daily before food for 15 days

Saraswatharishtam — 1.5 tablespoon twice daily after food for 30 days

Manasamithra vatakam   1 tablet with milk twice daily before food for 15 days

Mukta pishti   250 mg with clarified butter twice daily before food for 15 days

Mahakalyanaka ghritha   1 teaspoon with warm milk twice daily before food for 15 days

Brahmi ghritha   1 teaspoon with warm milk twice daily before food for 15 days

Chandanadi taila   for massage on the scalp

Himasagara taila   for massage on the scalp

Ksheerabala taila   for massage on the scalp

All of the above mentioned herbal formulations either single or in combination must be administered after a consultation with an Ayurvedic physician. The duration of the treatment may vary from patient to patient. Physician should decide the dosage and the duration of the therapy based on the clinical findings and response to therapy.

Chapter 8. Yogic Practices

The following yogic practices are beneficial in Anxiety, however, these should be performed only under the guidance of qualified Yoga instructor.

Duration should be decided by the Yoga therapist.
1. Pranayama (Breathing Exercise) Chandra bhedhi pranayama or the cooling Pranayama
2. Ujjayi - Ujjayi is a diaphragmatic breath, which first fills the lower belly (said to activate the first and second chakras), rises to the lower rib cage (said to correspond to the third and fourth chakras), and finally moves into the upper chest and throat.
3. Bhramari - Bhramari Pranayama, also known as Humming Bee Breath, is a very calm breathing practice that relaxes the nervous system and helps to be one with our inner nature.
4. Meditation along with the practice of Yama and Niyama.
5. Regular practice of Kunjal Kriya - Kunjal is one of the most effective yogic techniques. It is instantaneous in its action. It can give immediate relief to asthmatics and to those suffering from acidity, indigestion, headache, etc.
6. Jala neti- Jala neti, which is practiced using a neti pot filled with saline solution to cleanse the nasal passages. Here, the head is tilted to the side and then salt water is poured into one nostril and the water exits through the other one. This is one technique but there is a more advanced way where the water is poured into the mouth and snorted out the nose.

Chapter 9. Beneficial Yoga postures

Shashankasana or the Hare Posture

Sit in Vajrasana or the Thunderbolt pose . Place your hands on the thighs and breathe in a relaxed manner.

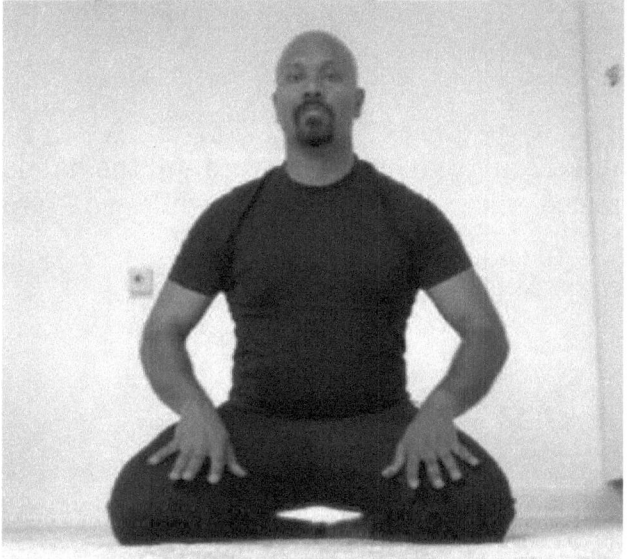

Raise both your hands above the head, palms facing forward. The arms should be in line with the shoulders.

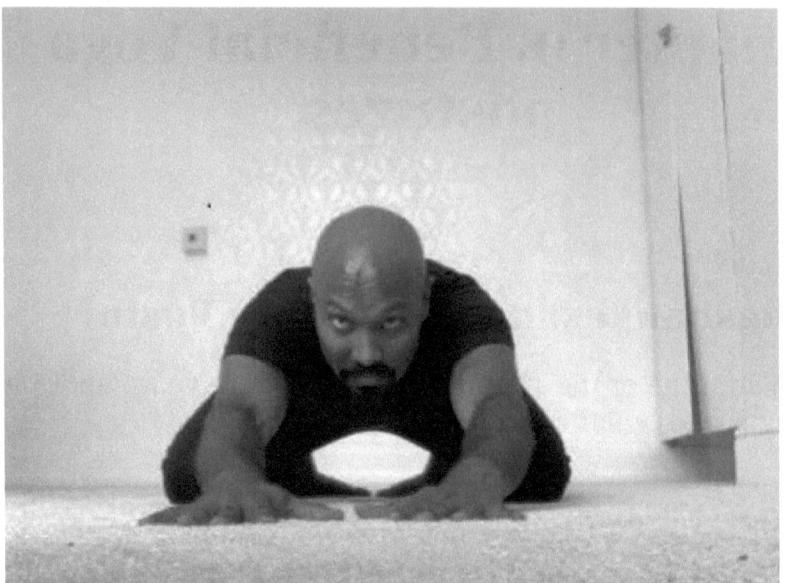

Slowly bend down and bring the hands forward, till the hands and forehead touched the ground. Exhale while you are bending forward.

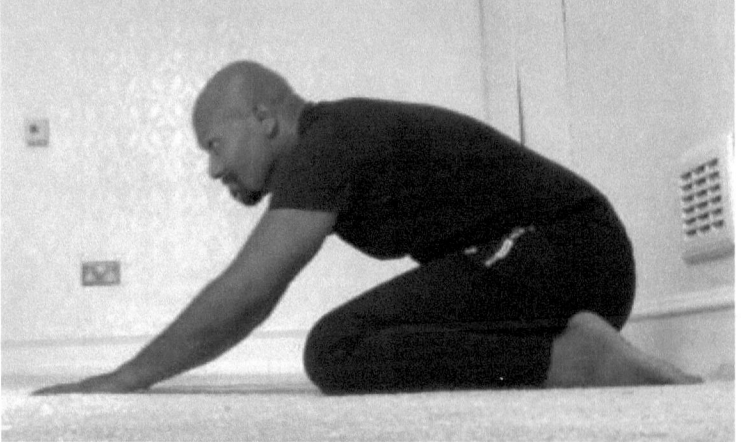

At the end, the forehead and hands rest on the ground. Rest in this position for as long as you are comfortable. Finally slow do rhythmic and relaxed breathing.

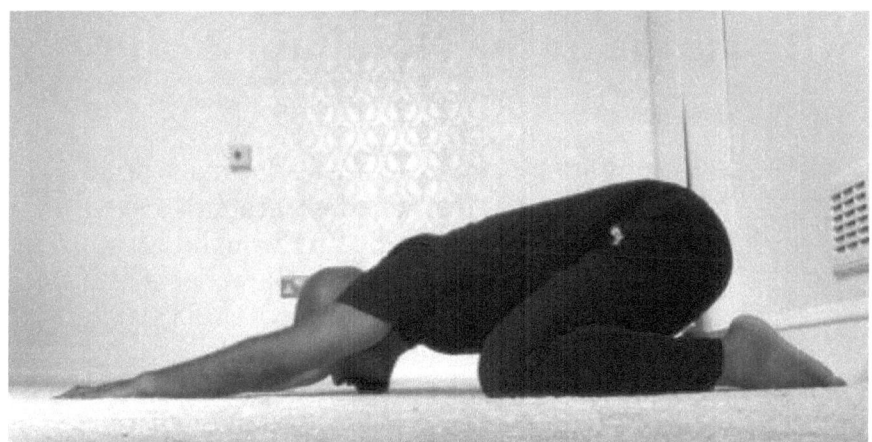

Exhale slowly and come back to the starting position. Repeat this twice or thrice focussing on the breathing.

Tadasana or the Mountain Posture

The mountain posture or the Tadasana is done standing with the feet together, grounded evenly through the feet and lifting up through the crown of the head. The thighs are lifted, the waist is lifted, and the spine is stretched upwards and straight with relaxed breathing

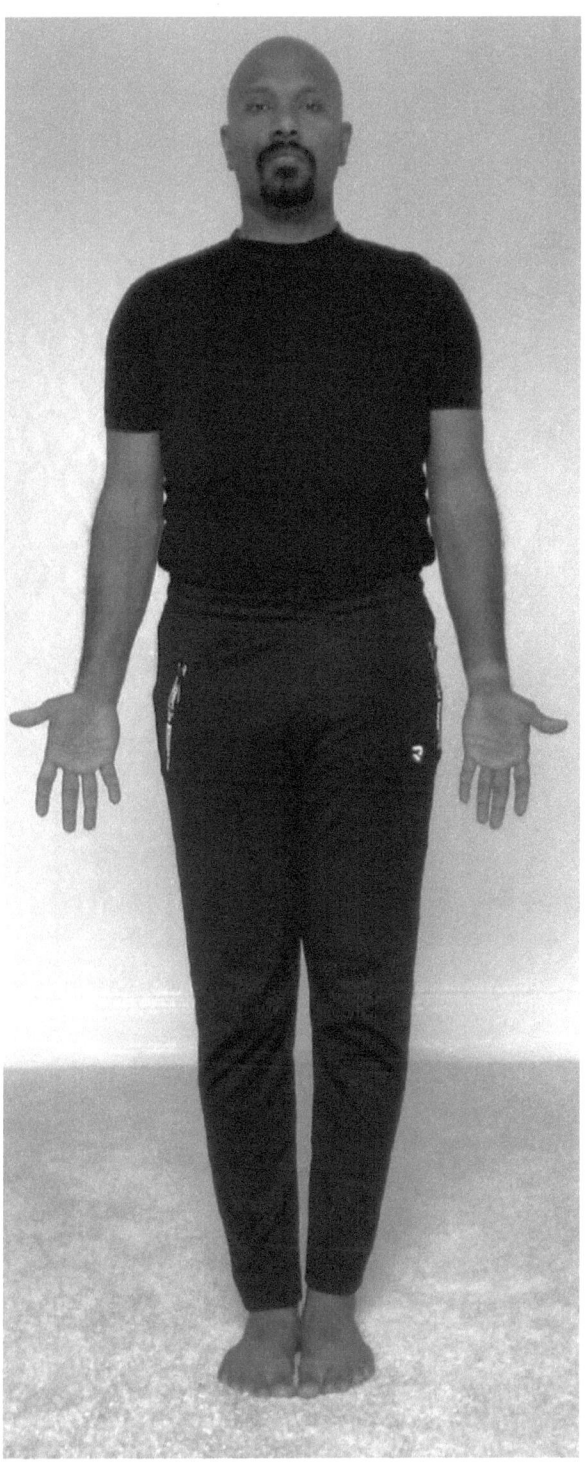

Anxiety Neurosis

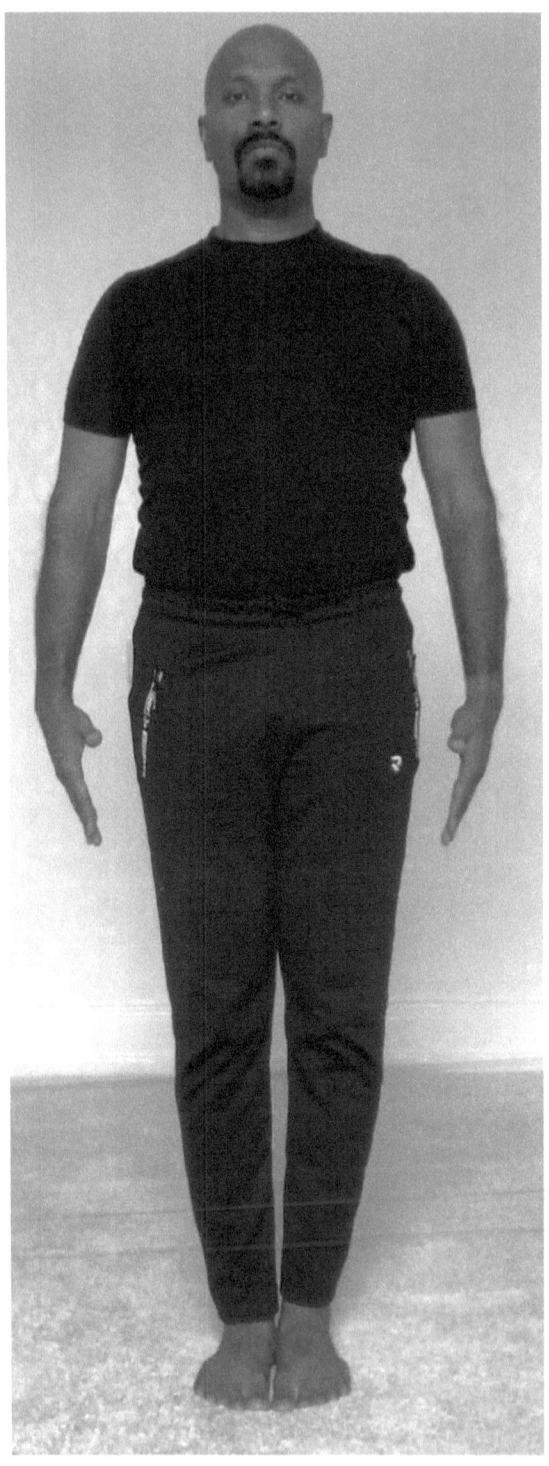

The mountain posture or the Tadasana is done standing with the feet together, grounded evenly through the feet and lifting up through the crown of the head. The thighs and the waist are lifted, and the spine is stretched upwards and straight with relaxed breathing

While the tadasana or the mountain pose, appears to be one of the most basic yoga poses, it is far more profound than it seems. Learning to tr stand in mountain pose, with awareness from the top of the head to the bottom of the feet, brings benefits in practicing nearly every other yoga pose — especially standing poses. Understanding the ins and outs of tadasana gives the knowledge needed to move confidently and safely into your practice for years to come. Regularly practicing mountain pose is also great for improving posture.

Matsyasana or the Fish Posture

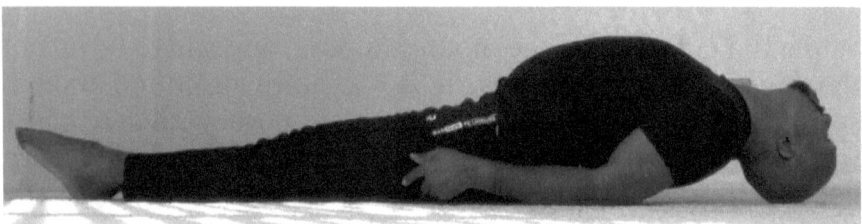

The Matsyasana or the Fish posture is a posture bending the back, the individual lies on his or her back and and the crown of the head is rested on the floor making the chest expand and protrude outward and upward. This gives a good stretch to the neck.

Mandukasana or the Frog Posture

Be seated comfortably in Vajrasana (thunderbolt Pose) with closed fists. Whilst clenching the fists press your thumb inside with the fingers.

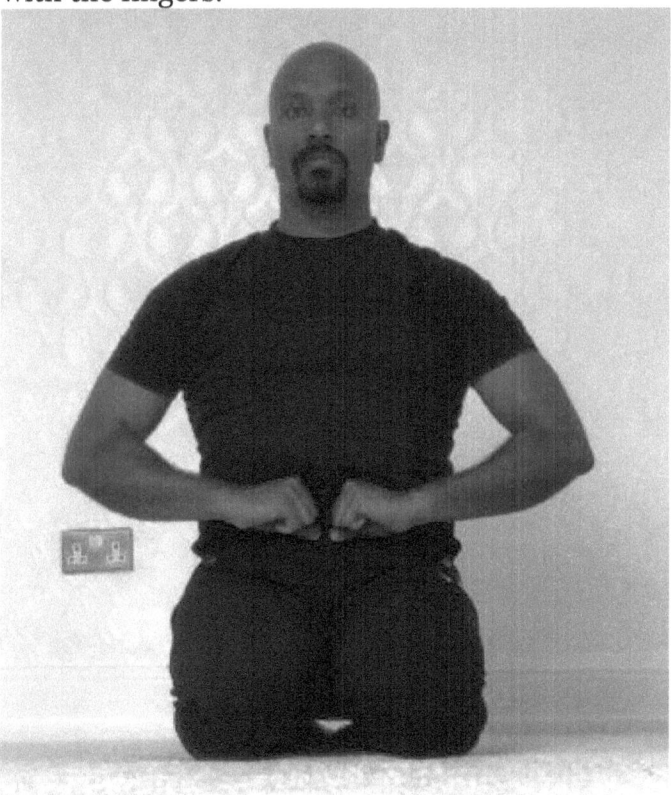

While pressing the navel with your both fists exhale and bend forward.

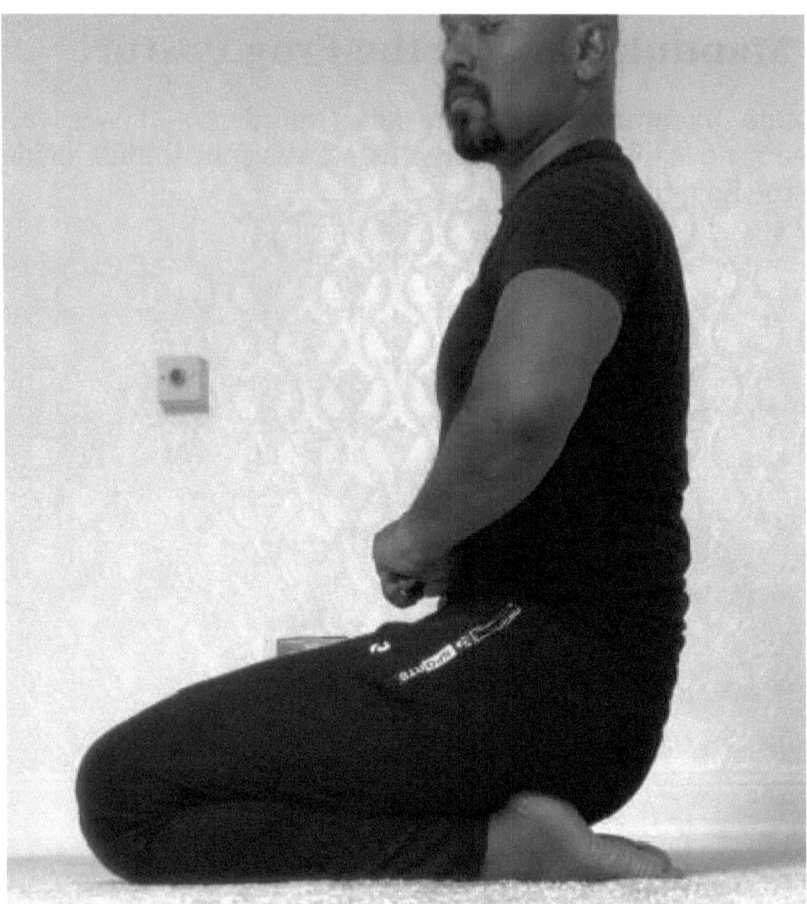

Hold the breath when you are in the position of bend forward and keep looking straight.

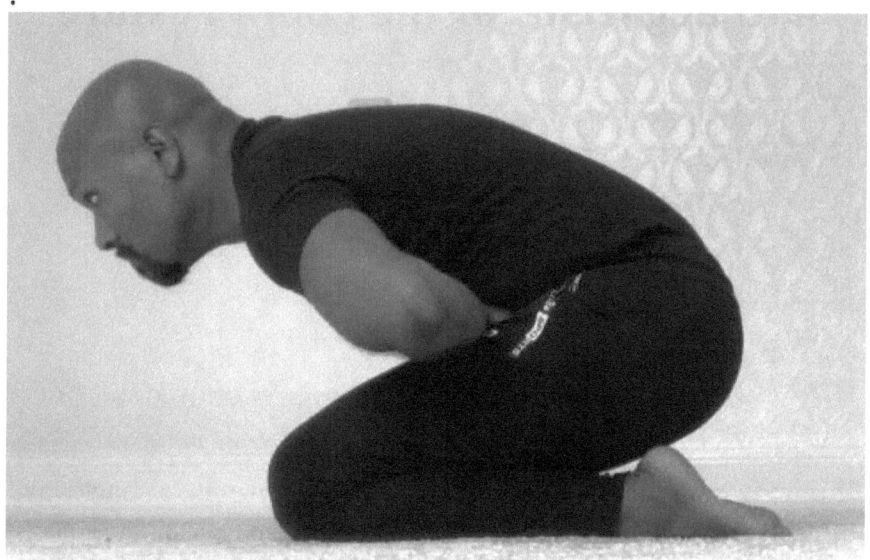

Stay in this position for some time as much as you can, inhale and come back to starting position (Vajrasana). Do this for 3 times.

Bhujangasana or the Cobra Posture

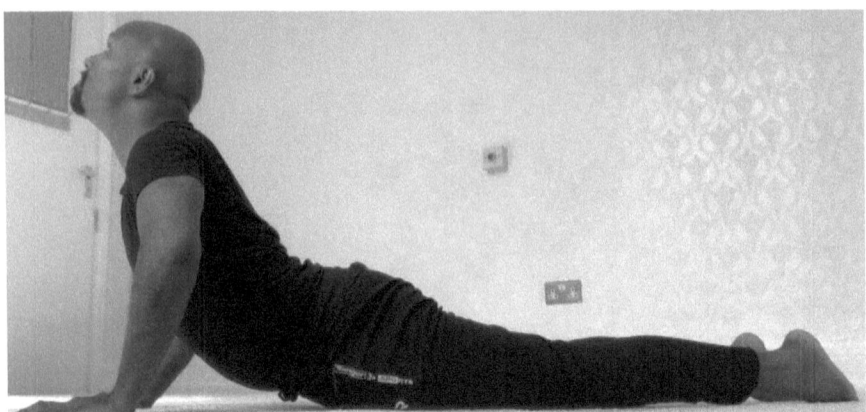

Bhujangasana also called as Cobra Posture is a backward bending pose. The Sanskrit name Bhujangasana is derived from two word. 'Bhujanga' stands for serpent while 'asana' means posture.

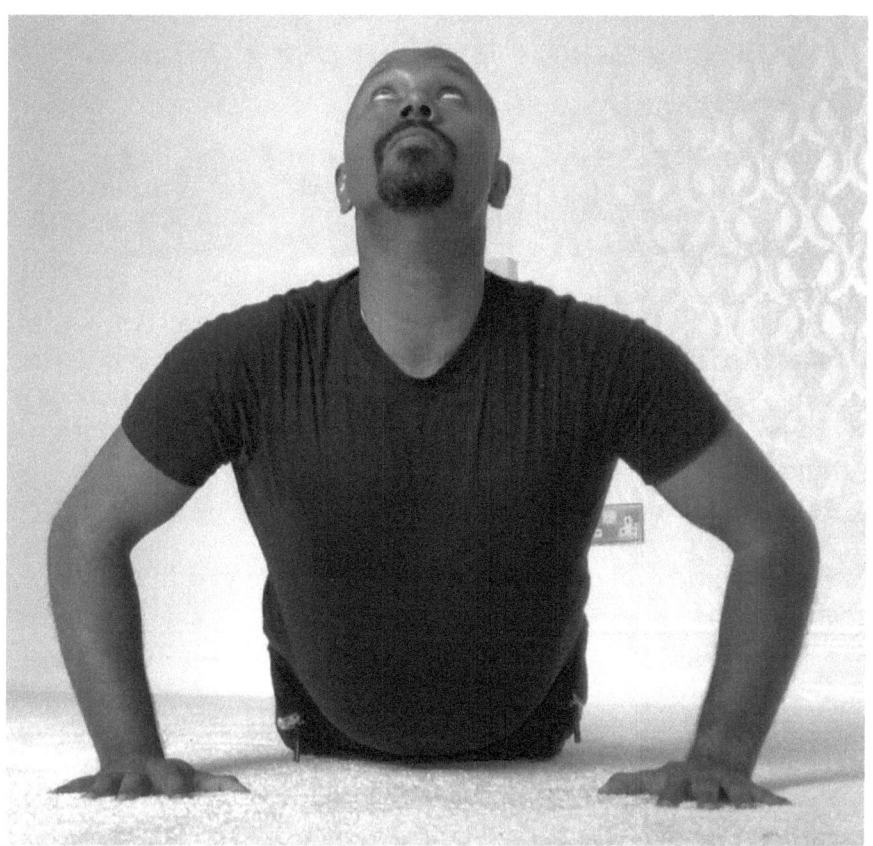

It resembles to the raised hood of a cobra. It is an excellent pose for strengthening spine along with many other benefits.

Shavasana or the Corpse Posture.

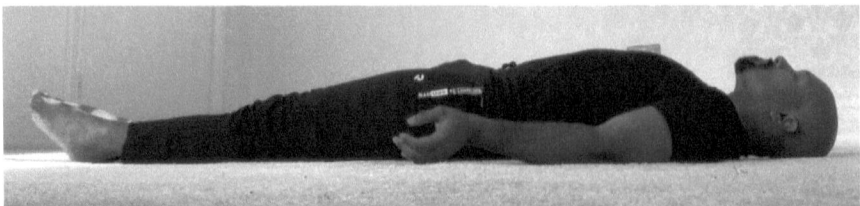

After doing all the above posture try and relax your body mind and soul for that inner peace and be one with yourself. Lying in this posture , concentrate in your breathing. Relax any strained part in your body by being in the posture for atleast 5minutes.

Some do's and don'ts that the individual have to adhere to on a regular basis-
1. Practice light physical activities, yoga and meditation
2. Read and listen to music
3. Avoid stressful conditions
4. Heavy meals at bed time
5. Avoid consumption of coffee, tea, soft drinks, alcohol and smoking

Yogic breathing is called Pranayama. Daily practice helps settle and calm your nervous system. Which is exactly what we need to do. There are many types of yogic breathing, Nadi Shodhan pranayama is supposed to be the best for anxiety. This incorporates the right and left brain settling the aggravated elements in the body and smoothing them. After this doing some meditation will be a bliss.

Intake of Vatha pacifying diet.
Intake of sugar is not healthy at all. Avoid caffeine, aerated drinks, cold/raw or frozen foods as you are trying to pacify vatha. Vatha dosha prefer salt, sour, sweet, oily and warm. Warm soups are helpful. Breakfast including oatmeal is good for settling anxiety. Also sweet fruits are good. Try and avoid ice water rather drink lukewarm water.

Avoid coffee, tea, cold drink and any energy drinks, reduce sugar and any type of chocolate.
Sleep enough at least 6 to8 hours, do regular exercise and meditation. Don't take much responsibility, as that can be a reason for stress.

In mental health, generally, anxiety is because of vatha vitiation, kapha aggravation is depicted by depression, and the anger is to do with the pitha vitiation.

Chapter 10. Important food that can help reduce anxiety

1. Brazil nuts-
Selenium has proven to be extremely effective in improving the mood in a person. Brazil nuts is rich in selenium, which help in improving the mood. Selenium also help in reducing the inflammation. Mushrooms and soybeans, are an excellent source of selenium. It also prevent cell damage. The anti-carcinogenic agent in it helps to prevent cancer from developing. Just keep it low in intake per day. Not recommended more than 3 brazil nut a day. They are also good source of Vitamin E. Low levels of vitamin E can also lead to depression and anxiety in some people.

2. Fatty fish
Omega-3 is a fatty acid that has a strong relationship with cognitive function as well as mental health.
Fatty fish, such as salmon, mackerel, sardines, and trout are high in
Omega-3. Often people eat other fatty acid called omega-6 instead of omega-3 and end up resulting in mood disorders. Its suggested eating at least two servings of fatty fish a week. Eating salmon three times a week reduces anxiety. Salmon and sardines are also among the few foods that contain vitamin D. Vitamin D deficiency could also lead to mood disorders, such as depression and anxiety

3. Eggs
Eggs contains all the essential amino acids the body needs for proper growth and development. An amino acid called tryptophan helps create serotonin. Serotonin is a chemical neurotransmitter that helps to regulate mood, sleep, memory, and behaviour. It also improve brain function and relieve anxiety. Egg yolks are another great source of vitamin D. It's an excellent source of protein.

4. Pumpkin seeds

Potassium regulate electrolyte balance and manage blood pressure. Pumpkin seeds are an excellent source of potassium. Pumpkin seeds and bananas are rich in potassium. It may help reduce symptoms of stress and anxiety. Zinc is essential for brain and nerve development and pumpkin seeds are also a good source of zinc.

5. Dark chocolate

Dark chocolate helps reduce stress and anxiety. Dark chocolate or cocoa can improve the mood. However, many of these studies are observational, so the results need to be interpreted with caution. They are rich source of polyphenols, especially flavonoids. Flavonoids inside our body can reduce neuro inflammation and cell death in the brain and it also improve the blood flow in our body especially inside the brain.

Like the eggs, the dark Chocolate are also high in tryptophan. Which the body uses to produce neurotransmitters, such as serotonin in the brain. Dark chocolate is also a good source of magnesium. A well planned diet with enough magnesium in it or taking supplements may reduce symptoms of depression and anxiety. Even though it's better than other chocolates, it still contain added sugars and fats, maximum 3gms is adequate.

6. Turmeric
The active ingredient in turmeric is called curcumin. Curcumin may help lower anxiety by reducing inflammation and oxidative stress that often increase in people experiencing mood disorders, such as anxiety and depression. An increase of curcumin in the diet reduces anxiety. Can add it with smoothies, curries, and anything really as it is okay in taste. It helps to boost your immune system. It is a powerful natural antibiotic.

7. Chamomile
Chamomile is known as the best herbal tea and is famous throughout the world. It is an ancient detox herb which is anti-inflammatory, antibacterial, antioxidant, and has muscle relaxant properties. The flavonoids present in chamomile makes it beneficial to combat anxiety.

8. Yogurt
Lactobacillus and Bifidobacterium are the two healthy bacteria present in the yoghurt. These bacteria and fermented products have positive effects on brain health. Yogurt produce an anti-inflammatory effect in the body. Chronic inflammation may be partly responsible for anxiety, stress, and depression. Consuming healthful bacteria keep the mind happy.

Including yogurt and other fermented food in the diet can benefit the natural gut bacteria and may reduce anxiety and stress.

Some of the Fermented foods namely are cheese, sauerkraut, kimchi, and fermented soy products.

9. Green tea
An amino acid called theanine, present in green tea has anti-anxiety and calming effects and may increase the production of serotonin and dopamine. Two cups of Green tea is highly recommended throughout the day, and replace soft drinks, coffee or any kind of alcoholic beverages.

Conclusion

Practicing yoga on a regular basis can help improve your overall well-being and may help manage your anxiety.

If you're new to yoga, talk to your doctor before adding this exercise to your routine. They can walk you through any potential risks and offer guidance on how to establish and maintain a healthy lifestyle.

If you'd prefer to practice at home, you can use books, articles, and guided online classes to develop your practice. Begin with a short practice of 10 minutes per day, and work your way up from there.
You can also take guided classes. Be sure to discuss your condition and intentions with your therapist so that they can develop a practice suited to your needs.

For those with depression adopting a regular yoga routine in addition to other healthy lifestyle habits can help over-come the condition.

It is always important to start with simple asanas. Avoid heavy exertion and instead focus on smooth, even stretch-ing and abdominal compressions. When beginning yoga, start with holding each posture for about five seconds, or as long as you are comfortable. As you progress, gradually in-crease the duration of each pose until you can comfortably hold asanas for up to one minute each.

www.ingramcontent.com/pod-product-compliance
Lightning Source LLC
Chambersburg PA
CBHW030740180526
45157CB00008BA/3250